Aphasia Readers Level 1

Aphasia Readers Level 1

A Day in the Life

Anna Teal

Illustrated by Austin Baechle

*This book is dedicated
with love and admiration
to my husband, Ryan.*

"And let endurance have its perfect result,
so that you may be perfect and complete,
lacking in nothing."

– James 1:4

BOOKLOGIX®
Alpharetta, GA

Copyright © 2022 by Aphasia Readers LLC

All rights reserved. No part of this book may be reproduced or transmitted in any form or by any means, electronic or mechanical, including photocopying, recording, or any information storage and retrieval system, without permission in writing from the author.

ISBN: 978-1-6653-0099-5

Printed in the United States of America   1 1 0 9 2 1

⊚This paper meets the requirements of ANSI/NISO Z39.48-1992 (Permanence of Paper)

Scripture quotations marked "NASB" are taken from the New American Standard Bible®, Copyright © 1960, 1962, 1963, 1968, 1971, 1972, 1973, 1975, 1977, 1995 by The Lockman Foundation. Used by permission.

Illustrations by Austin Baechle

Creamer illustration on page 6 by Denis Sazhin from the Noun Project
Tablet illustration on page 46 by Liam Mitchell from the Noun Project
Sleeve illustration on page 13 by Andrejs Kirma from the Noun Project
You illustration by Cuputo from the Noun Project

FOREWORD

When we are children, the importance of reading is drilled into us and reinforced by schoolwork and assignments. We tell children that reading is the door to other worlds. We tell them that they can fly to a freezing mountaintop in the oppressive heat of the summer or explore life in a rainforest while surrounded by concrete and millions of people in a city or meet fantastical beasts while safely tucked into bed. We tell them they can do this just by interpreting lines and letters on a page, digital or paper.

In more practical terms, we know that reading builds language and comprehension skills. It builds more empathetic people. It builds mental capacity and resilience. We know that reading lights up areas of the brain in a simulated experience. Read about a smell? Your brain responds as though smelling it. Read about a cool breeze on a stifling hot day? Your brain responds as though feeling it. Reading, particularly fiction and stories, can help us make sense of the world and understand where we fit in it.

Reading in a practical sense is also an important skill for communicating with others. Reading—and its converse, writing—is important for so many aspects of daily life, including filling out applications and other forms, reading instructions and learning a new skill, understanding emails from coworkers, or reviewing work products or concept papers developed by your team. So, when this skill is suddenly lost, as can occur with aphasia, it can have a very significant impact on your ability to interact with others, and your overall quality of life.

Aphasia is a loss of the ability to communicate through language. Imagine waking up one morning no longer able to say *hello* to friends or *I love you* to your family. You may struggle to understand what others are saying to you, and suddenly you are isolated from the rest of the world. Many people with aphasia also lose the ability to read and write. The impact of aphasia can be devastating, not just to the person who experiences it but also their entire family and social network, which can lead to mental health disorders and caregiver burden. Resources for treating and supporting people with aphasia are relatively scarce in this country, in part due to the lack of awareness of this disorder and the current unwillingness of insurance companies to pay for appropriate treatment. More tools are needed to help treat those with aphasia, and this book series is one important step in this fight.

Anna Teal—the author, editor, and driver of this aphasia reader—developed this book series to connect the magic and utility of reading that we experience in childhood—*but without making the reader feel like a child*. There is a vast distinction there. When someone has aphasia, their relationship with language and communication has inevitably changed. But it doesn't mean they have lost the fundamental ability to think or the desire to learn and experience through reading.

When Anna first proposed this book series, it was somewhat surprising in the sense that nothing like it really existed. With more than two million people in the US presumed to have aphasia—and thousands more who acquire it each year—how did we not have something like this available? There are beginner-level readers, of course, but they are often child-based storybooks that adults with aphasia have no choice but to use in order to practice their reading and pronunciation. As someone who may already be feeling disconnected from themselves and the life they were previously living, providing children's materials can be further isolating and demoralizing.

Anna proposed a system that could significantly impact the field of aphasia care for adults. The reader would still be easy to understand with images throughout to maintain interest and to provide cues to the reading passages but the stories and content would be more adult-oriented. When she brought this to our program, the University Center for Language and Literacy at the University of Michigan, we knew it was something we both wanted and needed to be involved with. As leaders in aphasia treatment through our intensive University of Michigan Aphasia Program (UMAP), as well as our expertise in reading and literacy through our Reading Intervention Program, we were also uniquely qualified to help her bring the concept to life.

What you will read in the coming pages is just that: the heart and vision of one very dedicated person, Anna, partnered with the professional backing of our team of language and literary experts. This project brings the community, faculty, and our experts in the field together, to accomplish important change in the way people with aphasia are treated and the high-quality resources they have available.

To those in the aphasia community, we hope this reader says: you are not alone, and you do have a voice. It may sound different than before, but there are people out there who are listening. We thank you for this opportunity to better understand what you need and how we can serve you. Our UMAP program began more than eighty years ago with the aim of giving compassionate and individualized care to people with aphasia, to providing them with hope and practical tools to move forward. This book is another step in that direction.

Carol Persad, PhD, ABPP-CN
Clinical Professor
Director, University Center for Language and Literacy, Mary A. Rackham Institute
Director, Neuropsychology Program, Department of Psychiatry
University of Michigan and Michigan Medicine

PREFACE

Aphasia Readers was created by husband-and-wife team, Ryan and Anna Teal. Ryan had a massive stroke at the age of thirty-four which left him with aphasia and apraxia. Throughout his recovery, the repetition of reading aloud seemed to be a tried-and-true form of speech practice with promising results. However, the only books available to practice on a simple level were children's books. As an adult, reading these types of books felt a little demeaning. Although Ryan and Anna had many good laughs reading about "a trip to grandma's house," they quickly realized a need for simple, short readers with adult-themed content to support those in the aphasia community.

After more than a year in the making, and extensive collaboration with the renowned University of Michigan Aphasia Program at the University Center for Language and Literacy and input from top neurological teams, they finally wrote their first book of *Aphasia Readers* for adults. Their ultimate hope is to provide accessible and affordable supplementary speech practice tools for others in the aphasia community that will help pave the way for a successful recovery. A portion of the proceeds from each book goes back into supporting aphasia awareness and helps others pay for much-needed intensive speech therapy.

INTRODUCTION

Aphasia Readers: Level 1 is a supplementary recovery tool for adults with Aphasia who want to practice reading aloud to improve their speech. *Level 1* is designed to be a base-level practice, with mostly one-syllable words. This book has six total themes designed to relate to a person who is early on in their recovery.

There are multiple ways to use this book:

- Practice by yourself.
- Practice the dialogue with a loved one, friend, or caregiver.
- At the end of each section, you'll find customizable pages to utilize outside of practice. You'll also find detailed pictures that give you plenty to describe to help with writing practice.
- In each sentence, there are pictures associated with certain words. This is to help with word retrieval in case you get stuck.
- Feel free to read one section a day, or if you're having a good day, read multiple sections to build on your practice.
- Don't forget to recall your practice sentences throughout your day-to-day activities.
- Visit our website at www.aphasiareaders.com for FREE, downloadable practice worksheets.

These readers were thoughtfully designed with a spiral-bound structure so those with a weaker side can manage the workbook comfortably. We know those with aphasia can get overwhelmed quickly, so all illustrations were created with calming, soothing colors to help you feel at ease while you practice.

TIP: If you're reading aloud by yourself, use a speech-to-text app to check your pronunciation.

Session 1

A Good Morning

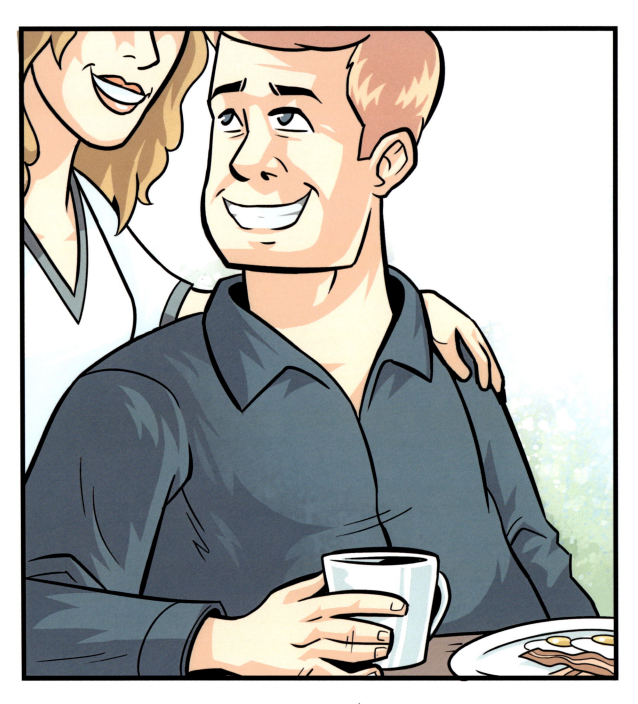

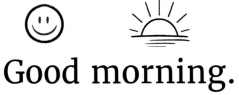

Good morning.

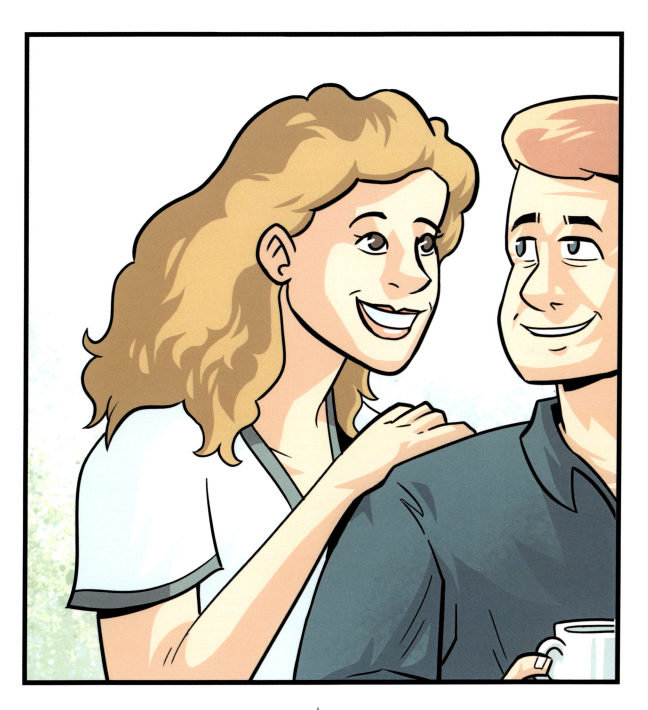

Good morning, love.

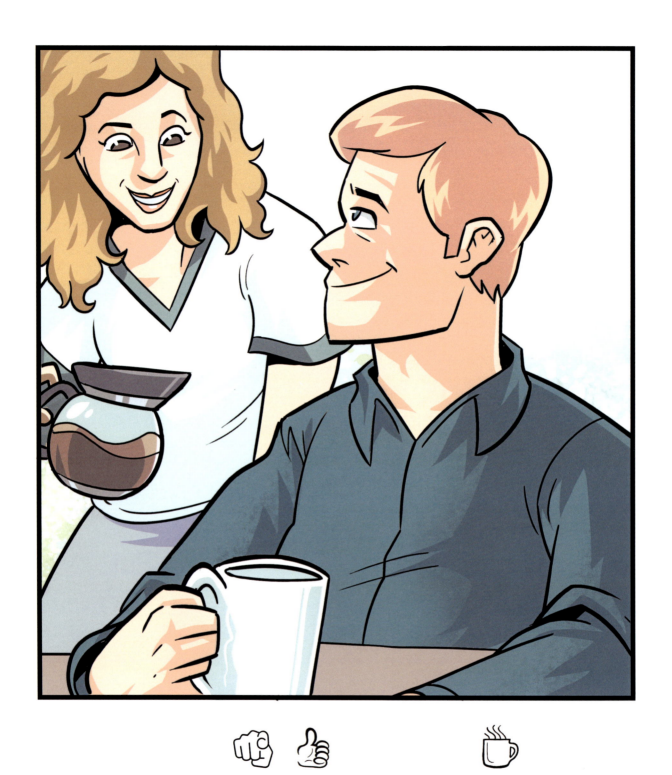

Would you like more coffee?

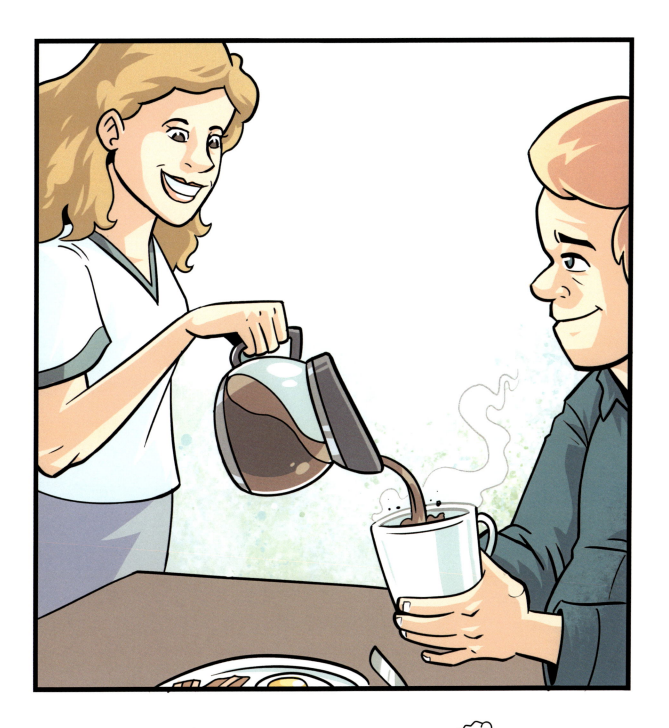

Yes, please. Thank you.

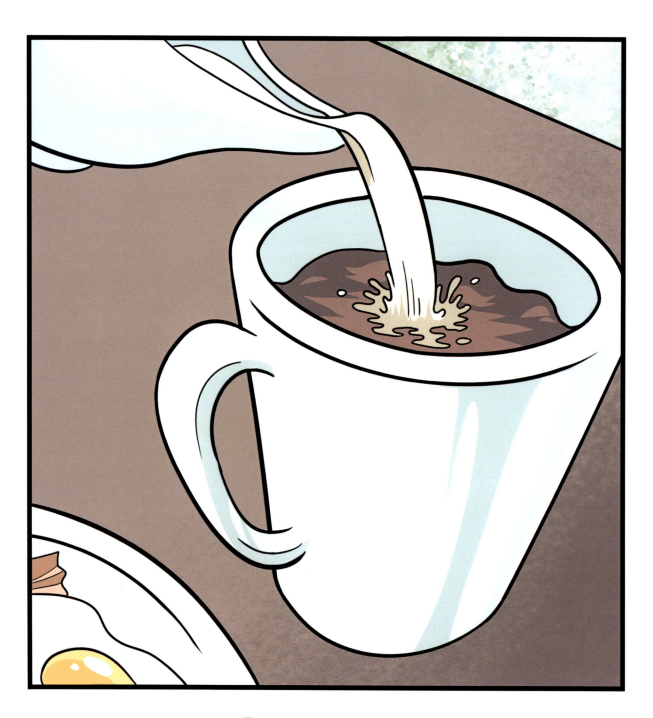

Creamer? Yes, please.

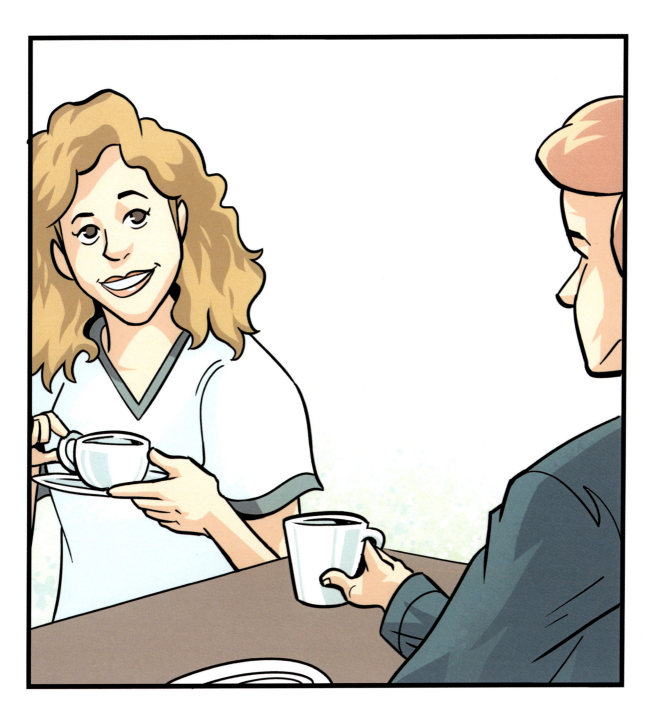

Today will be a good day.

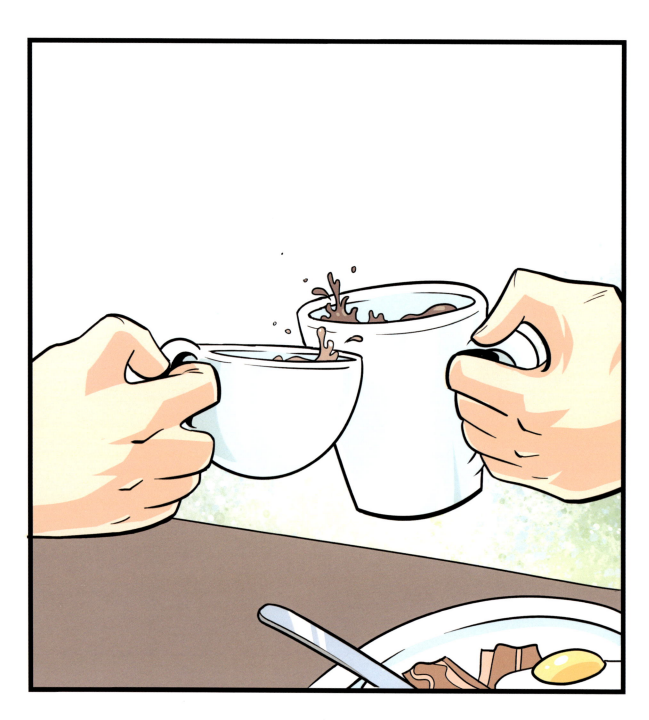

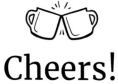

Cheers!

Customize and Practice Your Order

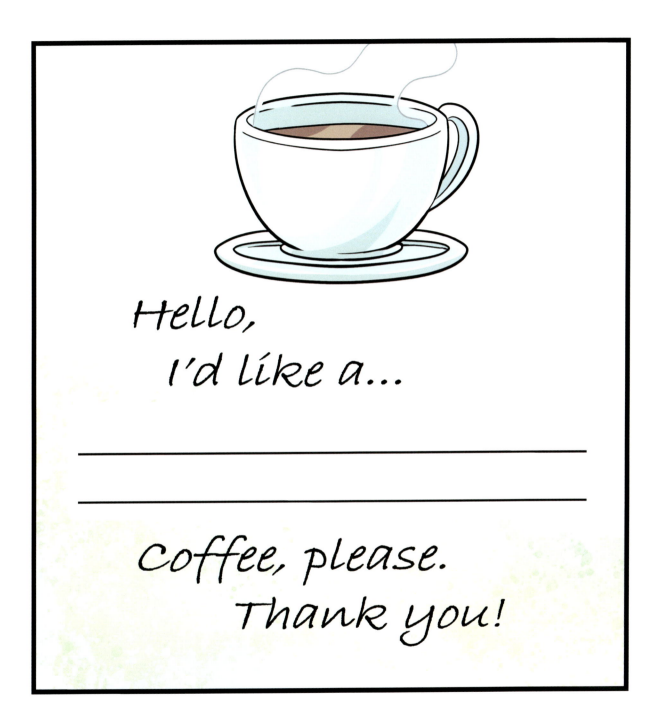

Notes

Session 2

Dressed to Impress

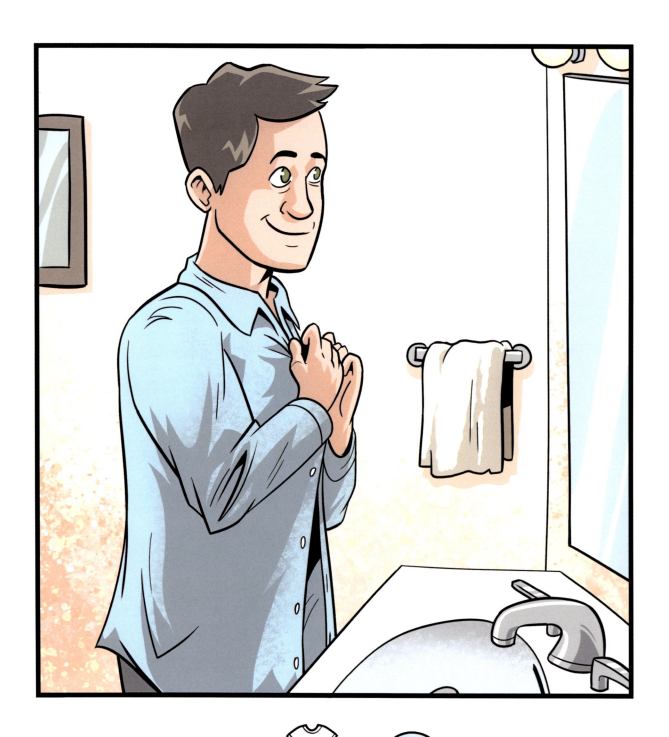

My shirt is blue.

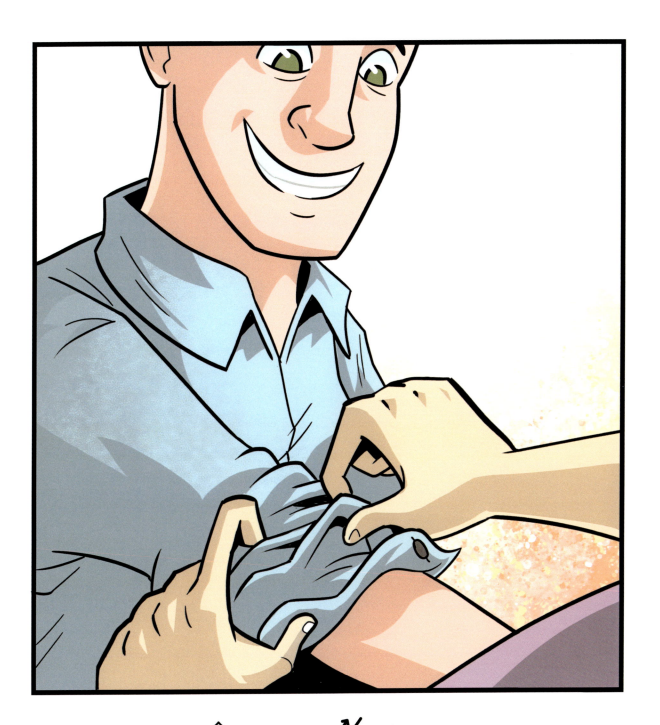

Roll up my sleeve, please.

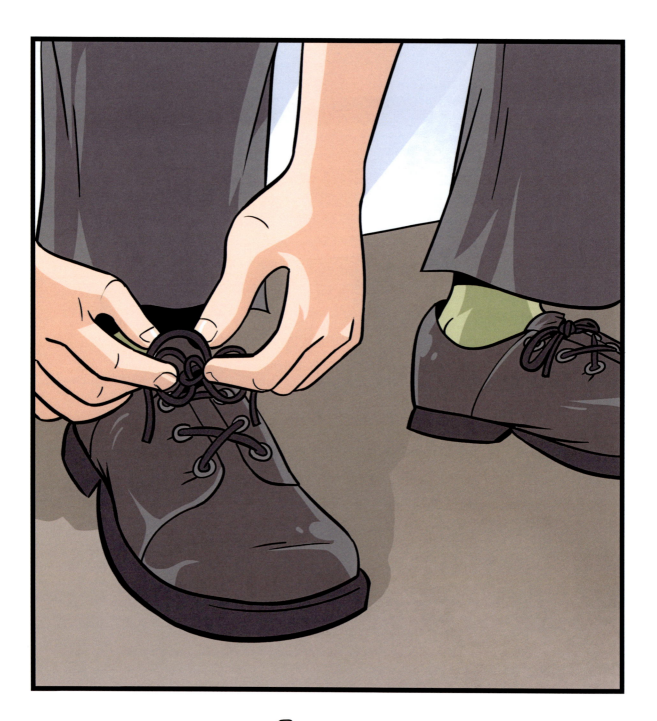

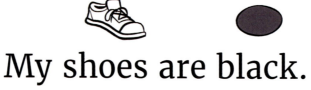

My shoes are black.

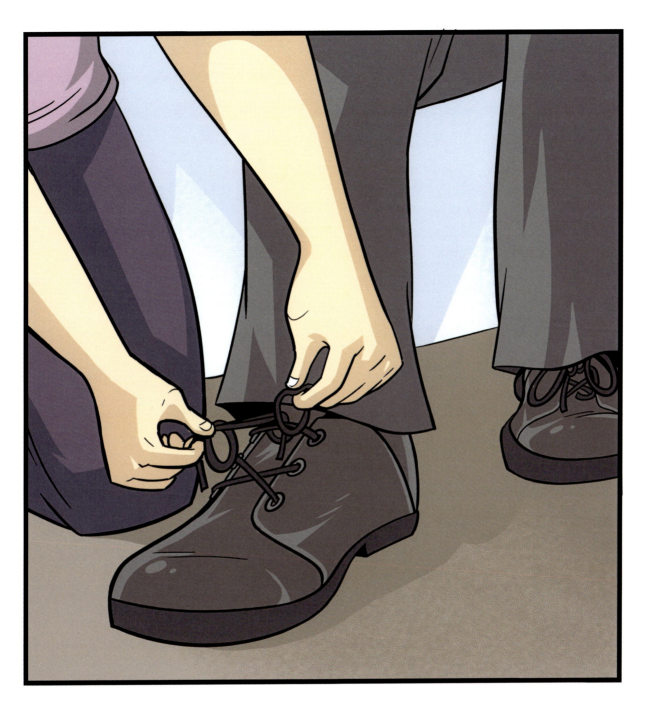

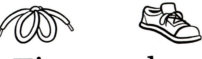

Tie my shoe, please.

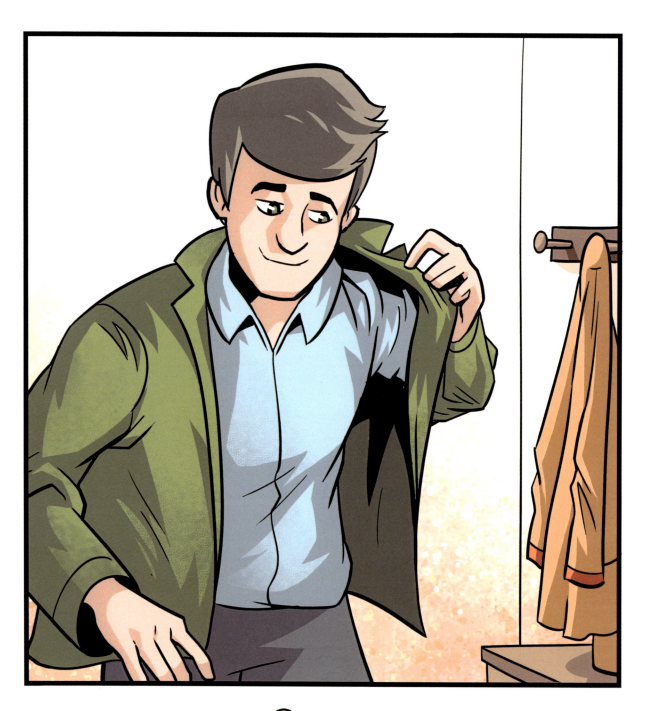

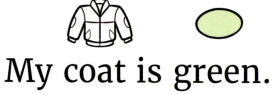

My coat is green.

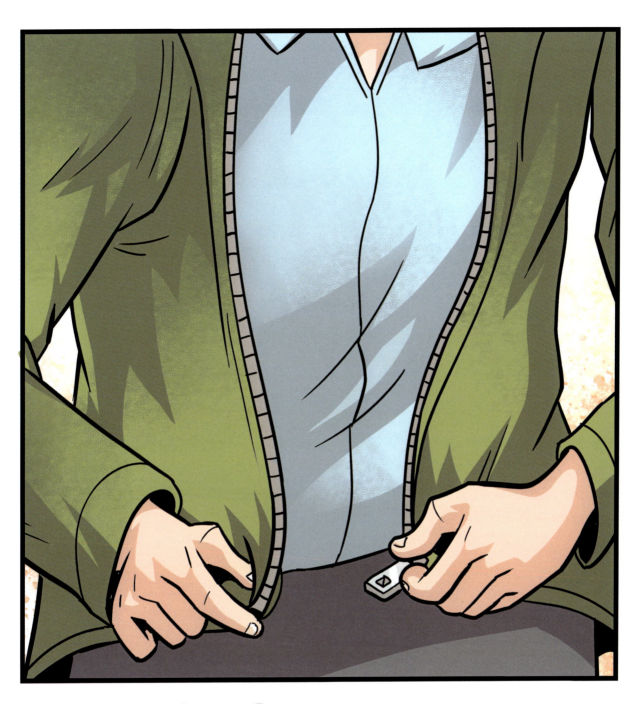

Zip me up, please.

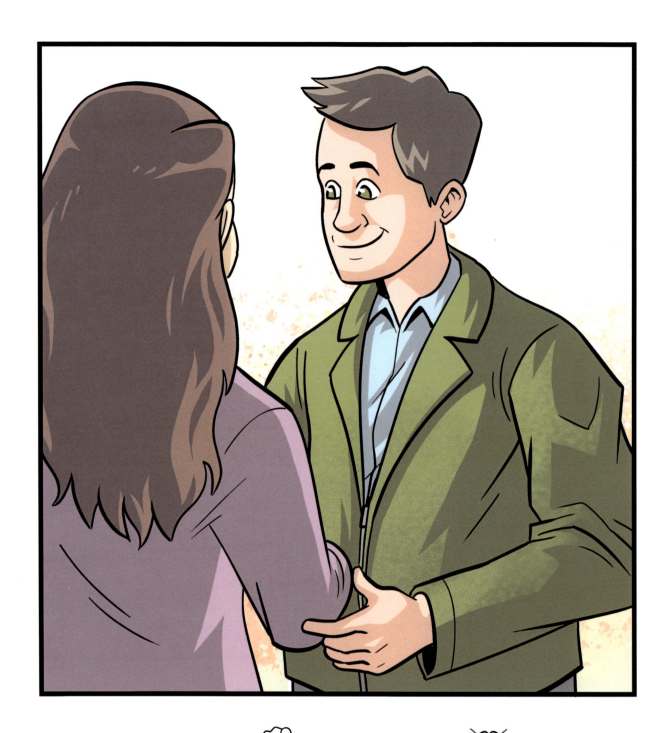

Thank you for your help.

Write About What You See

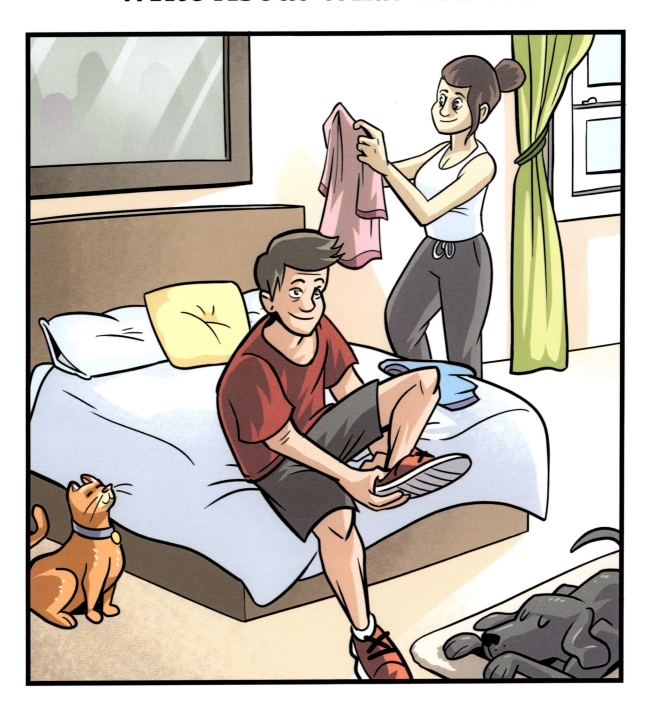

Notes

Session 3

Pets

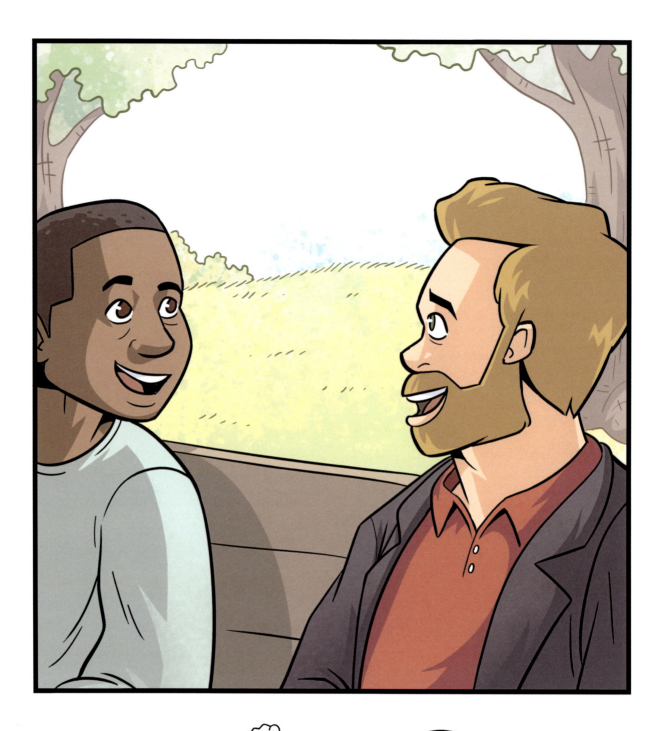

Do you have a pet?

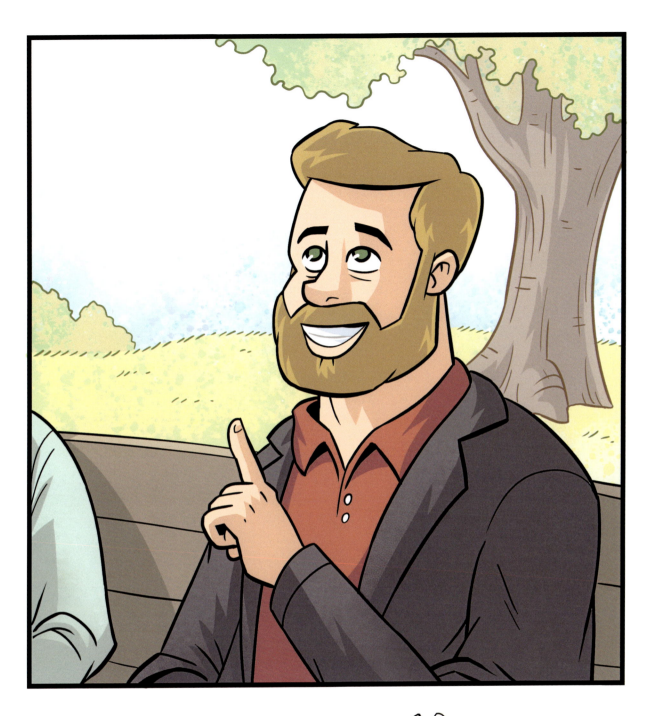

Yes, I have a dog.

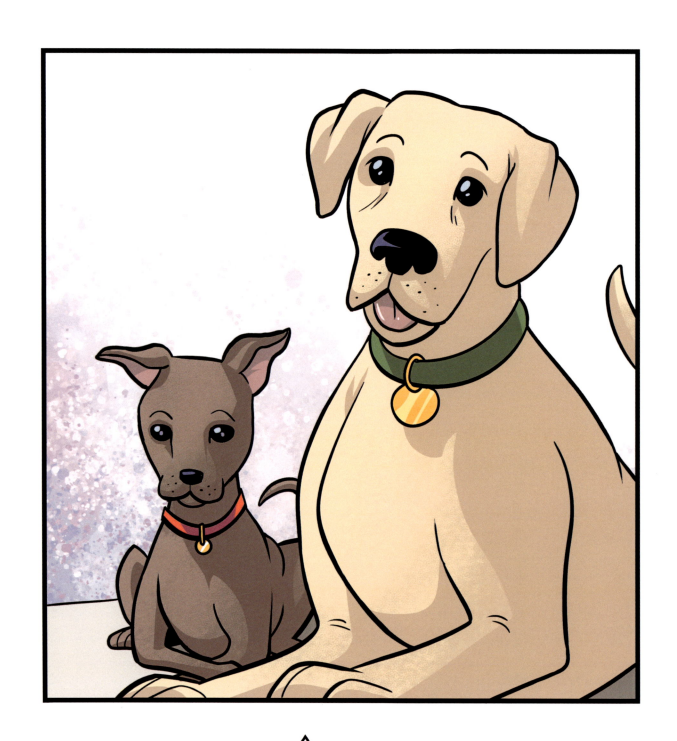

Is he big or small?

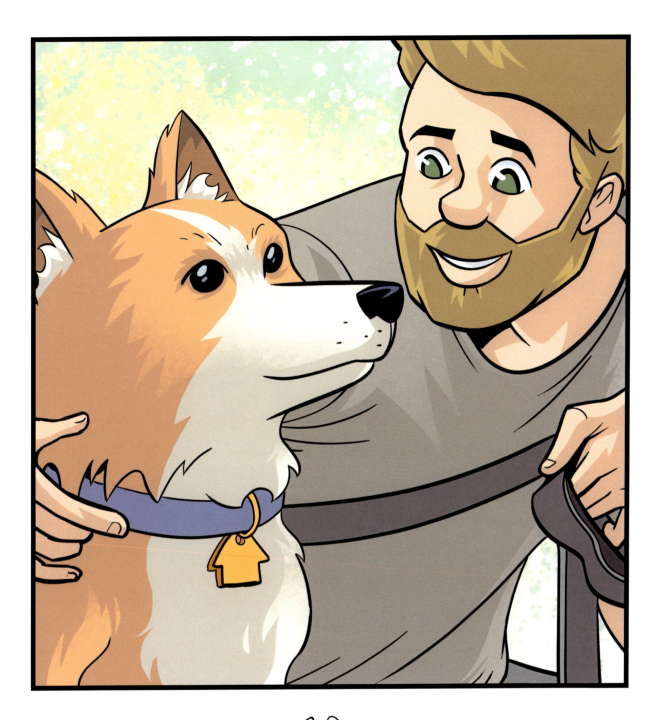

△ 🐕

He's a big dog named Ted.

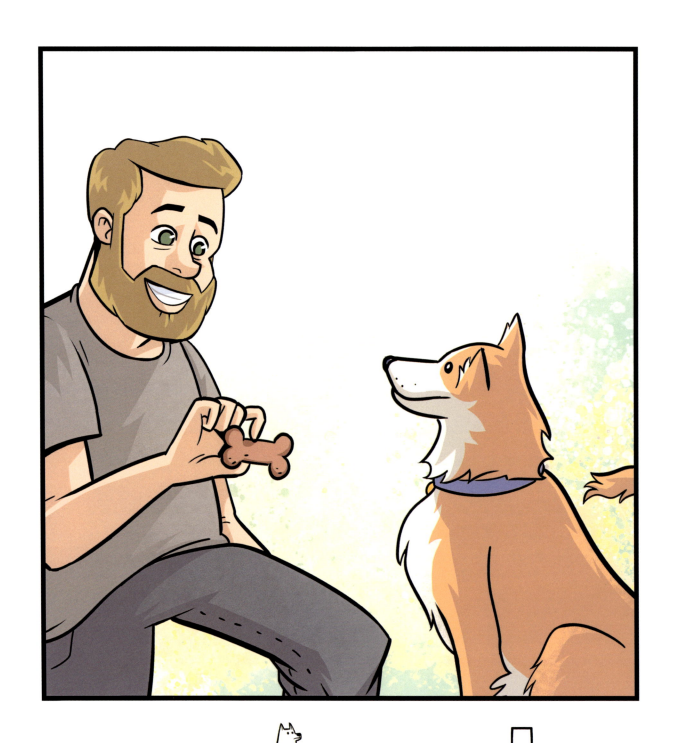

He knows sit, stay, and down.

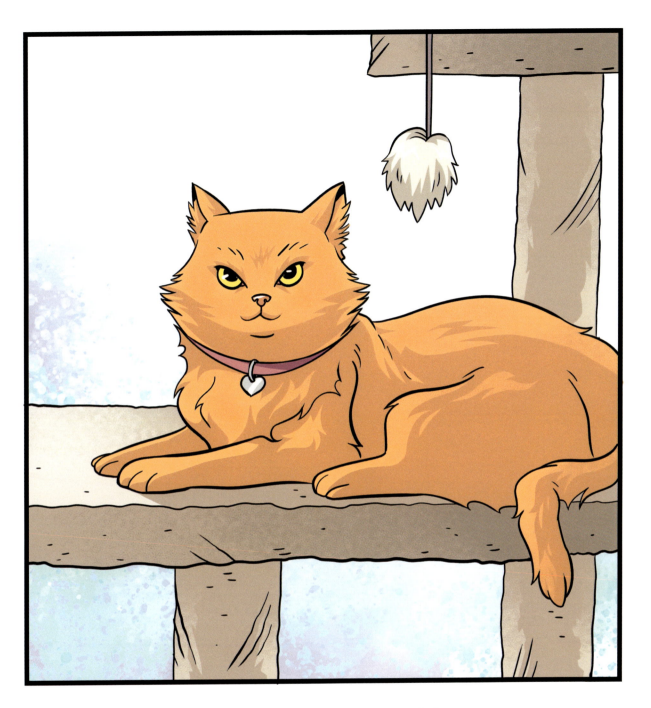

What about a cat?

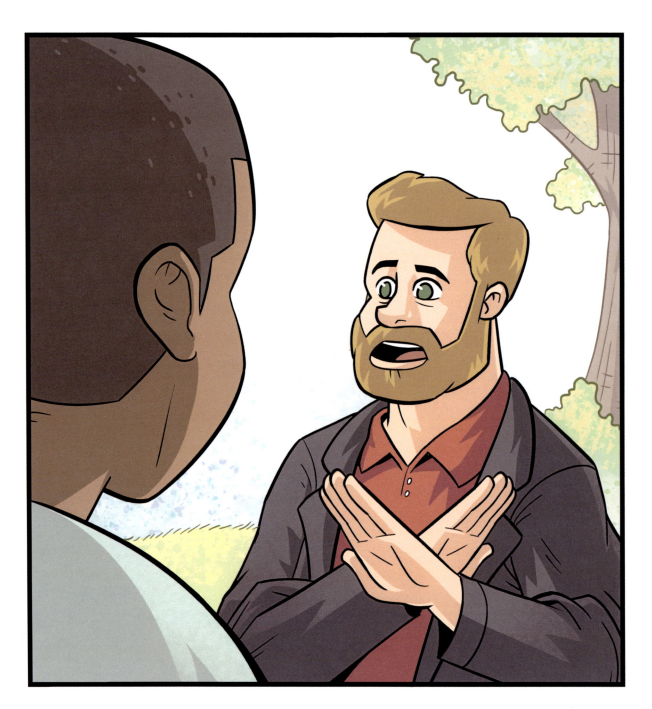

No! I don't have a cat.

Write About What You See

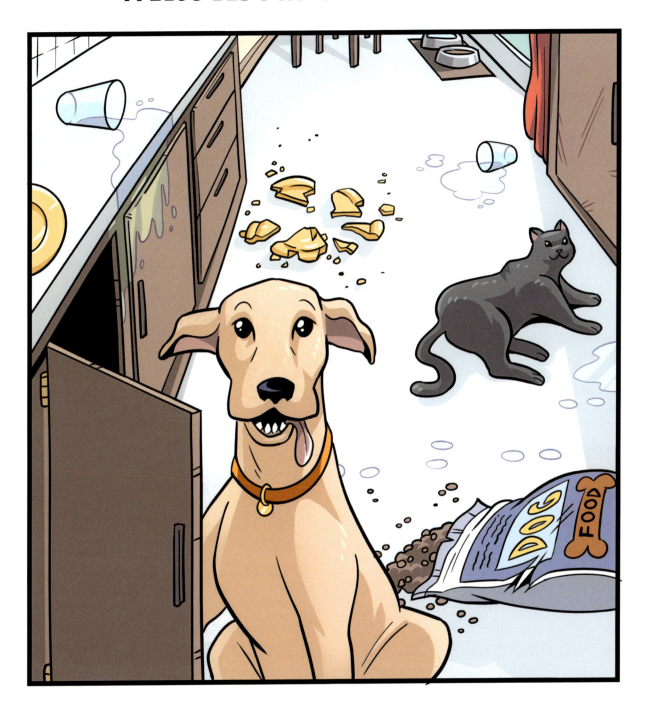

Notes

Session 4

Walk in
the Park

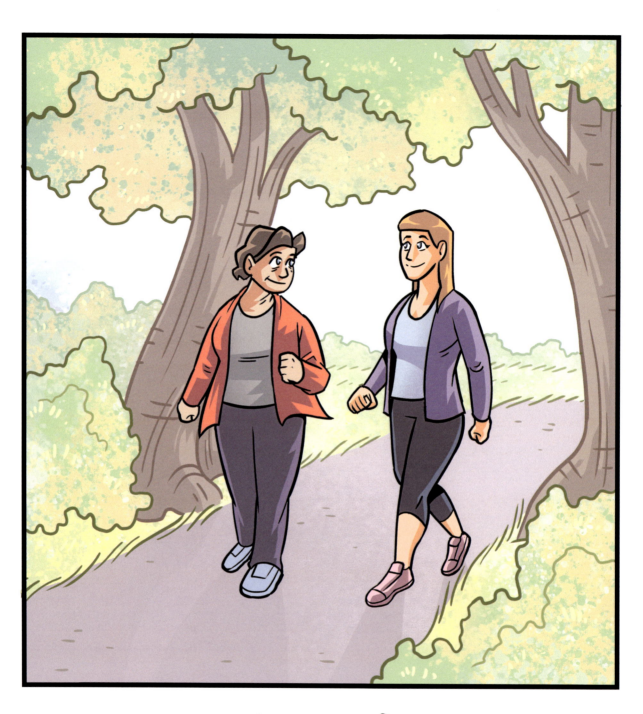

I like to walk.

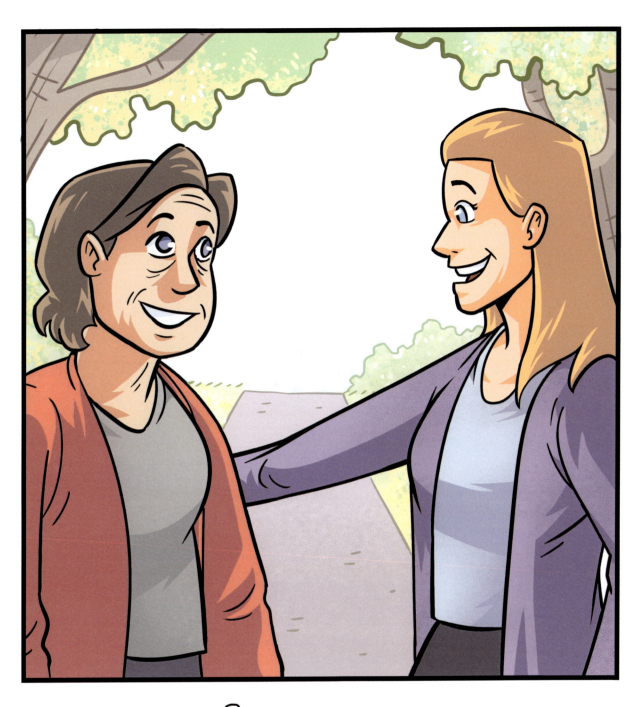

Me too, Mom.

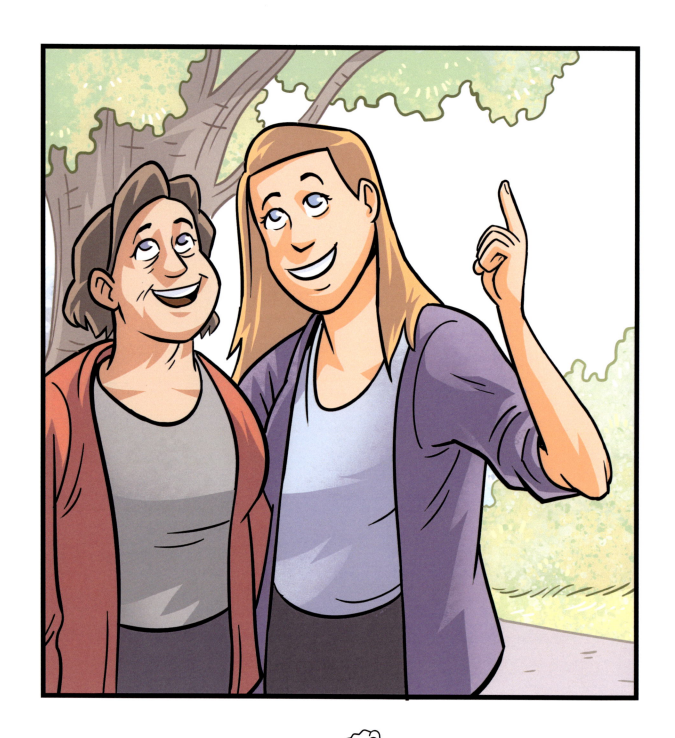

What do you see?

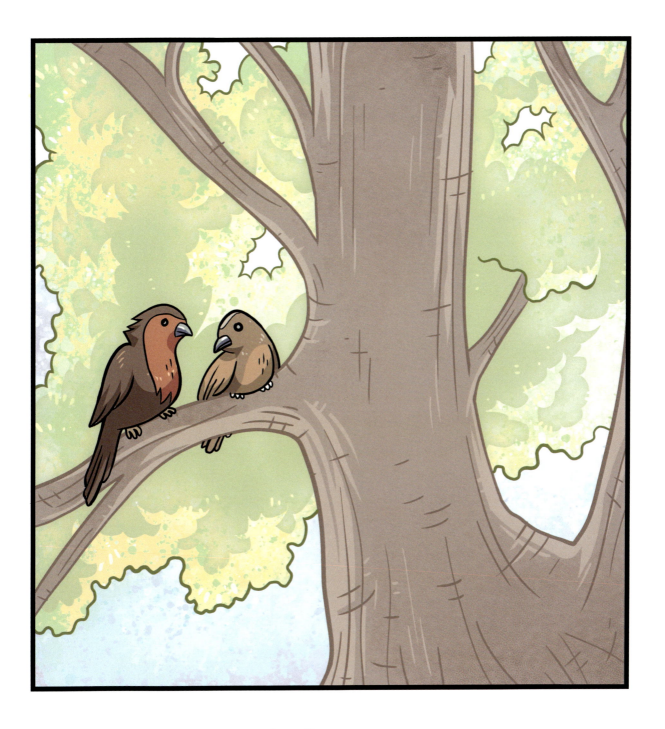

I see trees and birds.

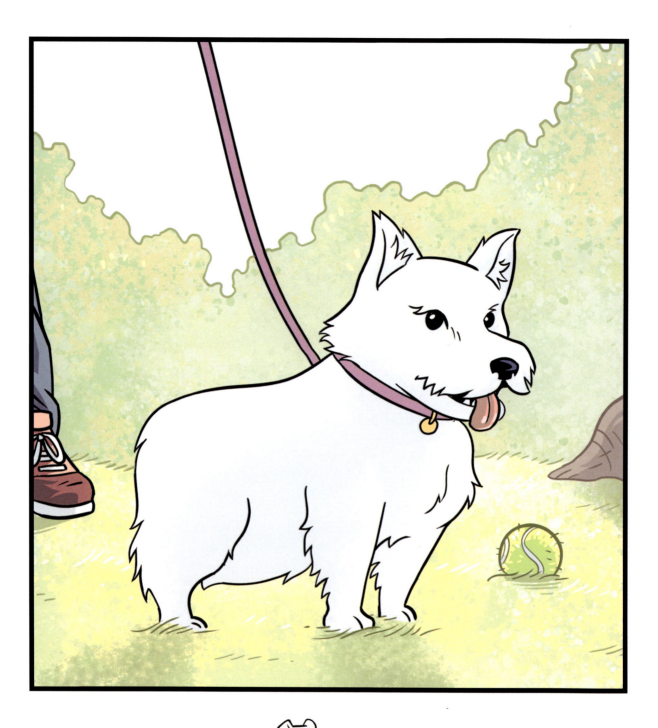

I see a dog and grass.

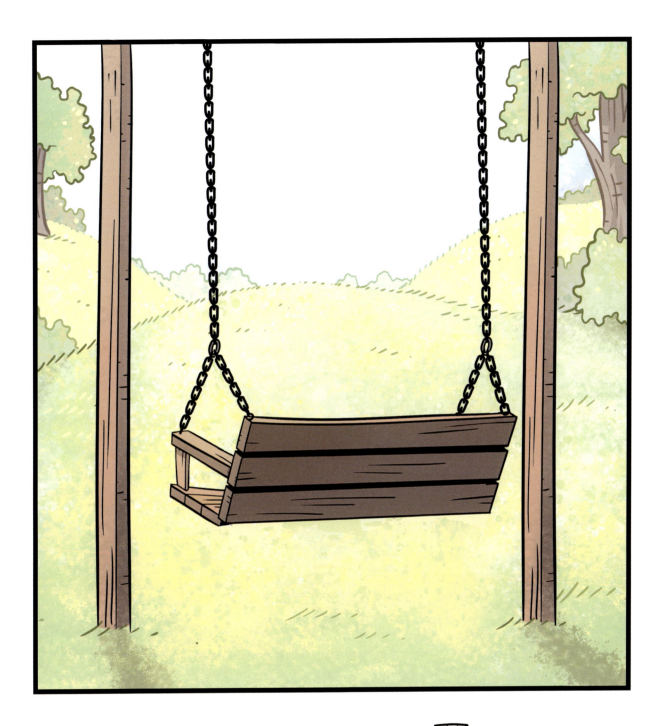

I see hills and a swing.

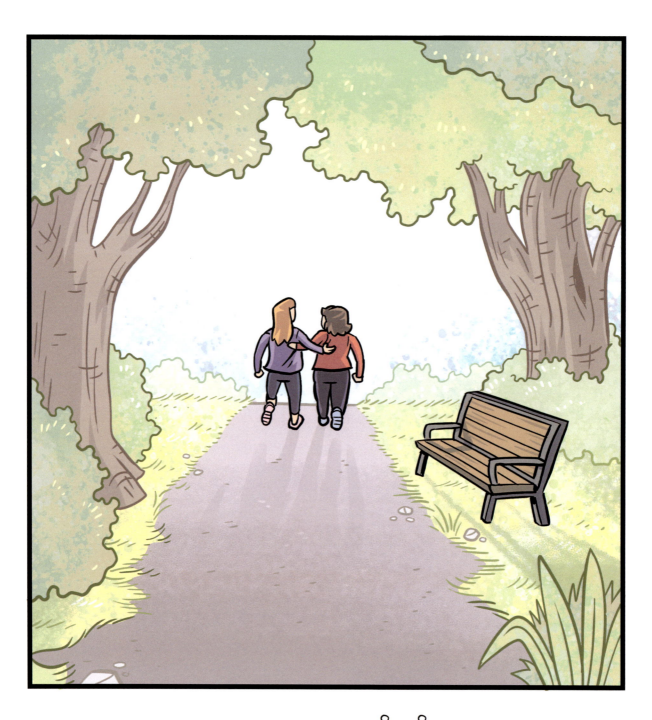

I love our walks.

Write About What You See

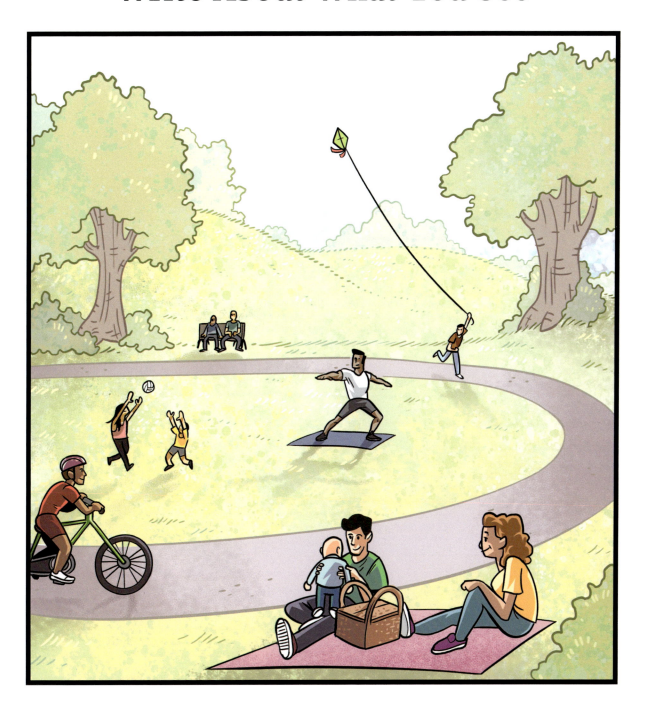

Notes

Session 5

Tech Talk

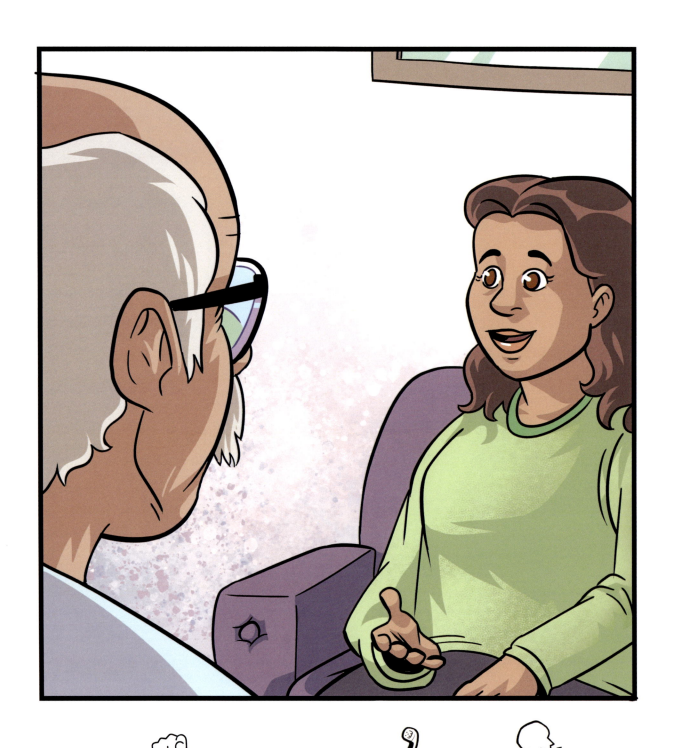

Do you use your phone to talk?

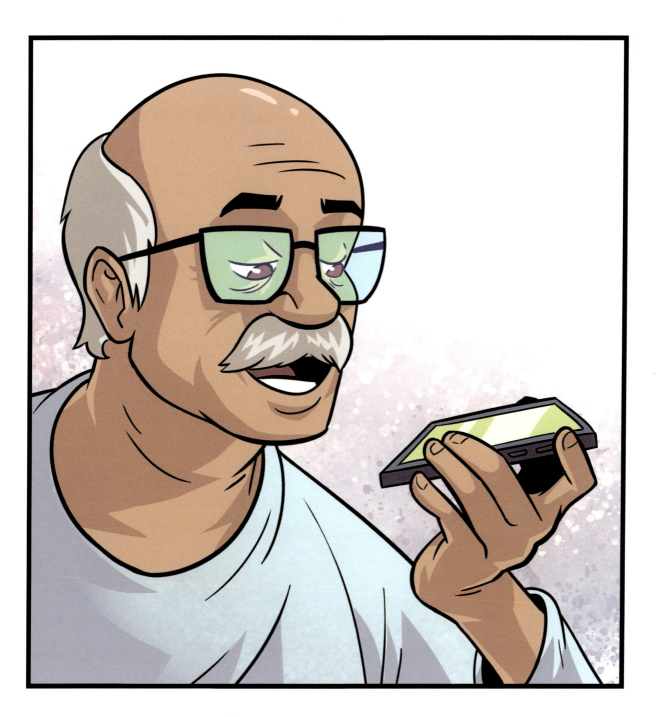

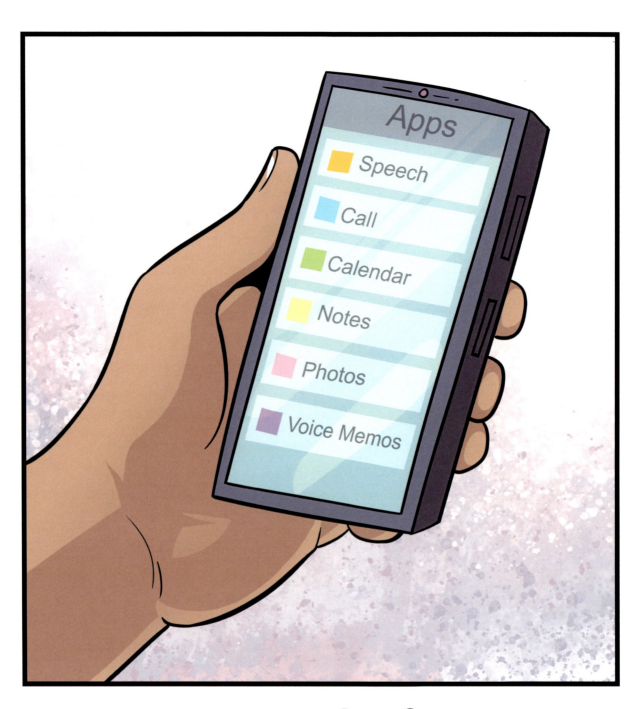

It helps me talk.

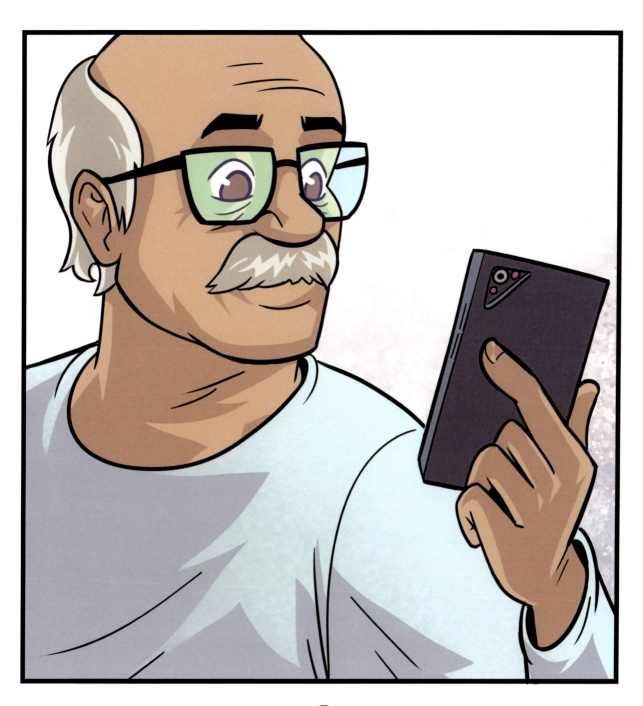

It helps me listen.

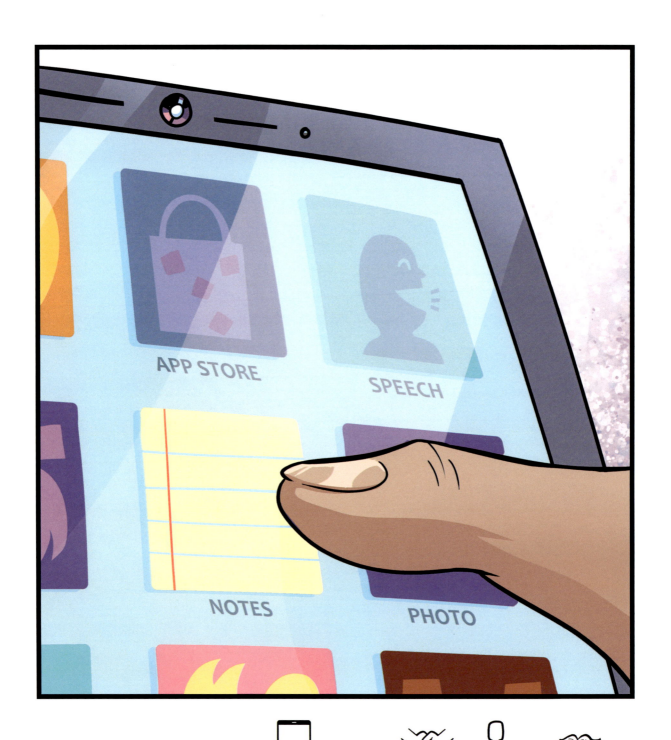

I also have a tablet to help me learn.

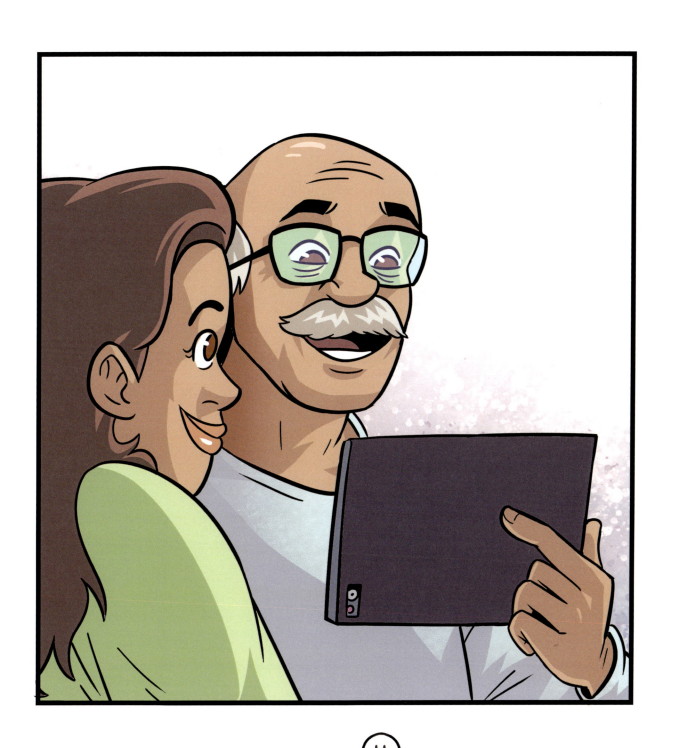

🙂

It's a very good tool.

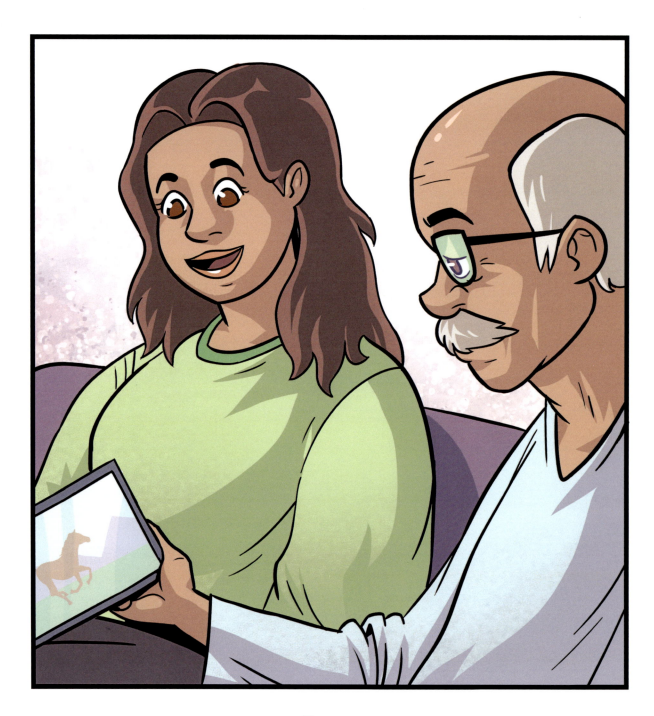

☺

That's good to know.

Write About What You See

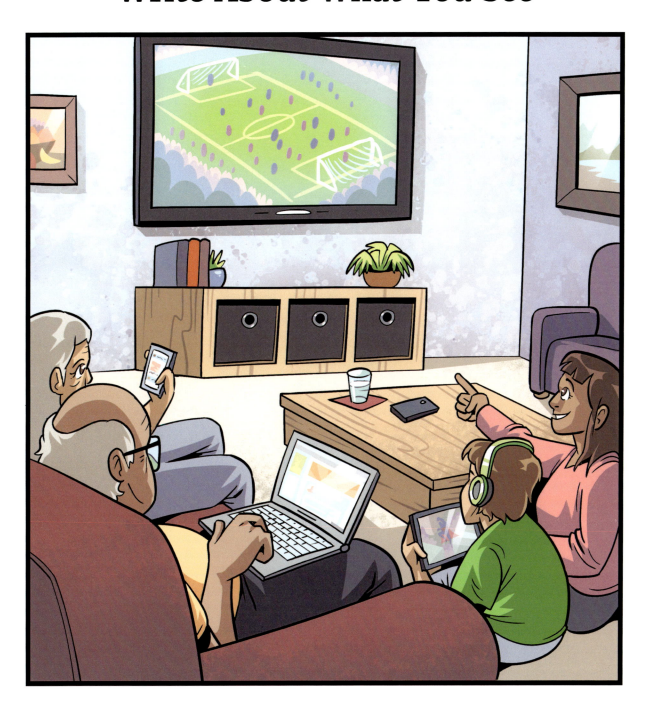

Notes

Session 6

Ordering Out

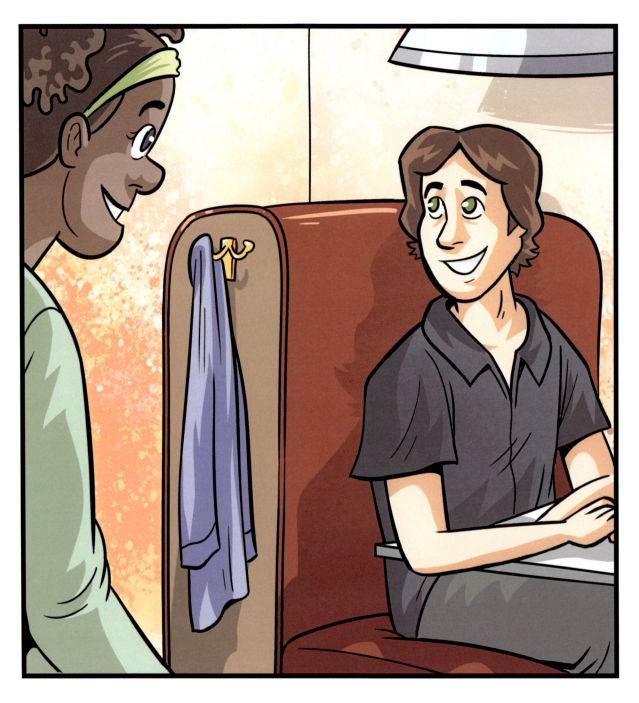

Hello, what would you like to drink?

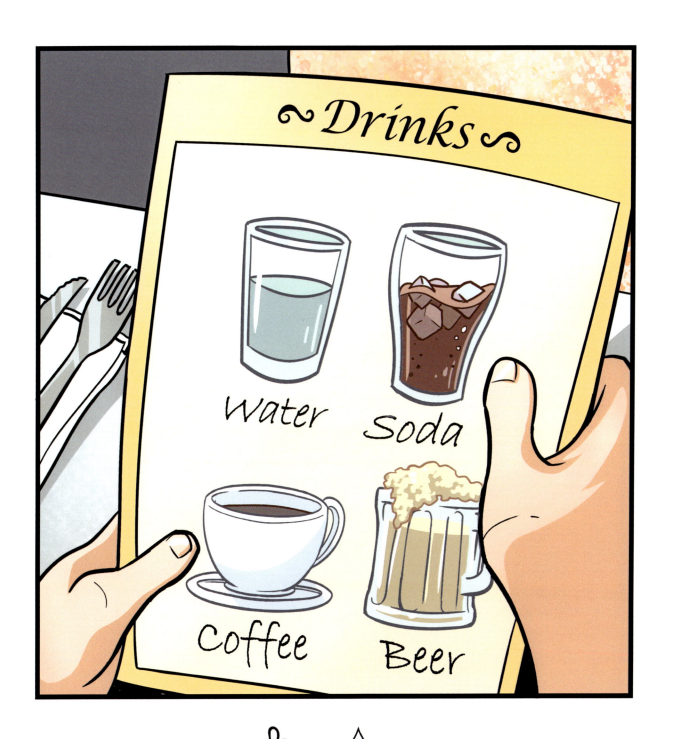

Hi, I'd like water, please.

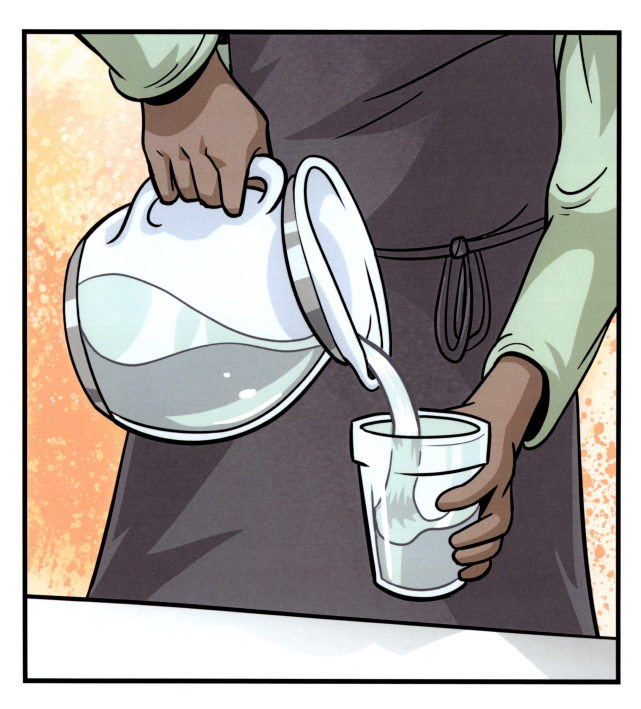

You got it!

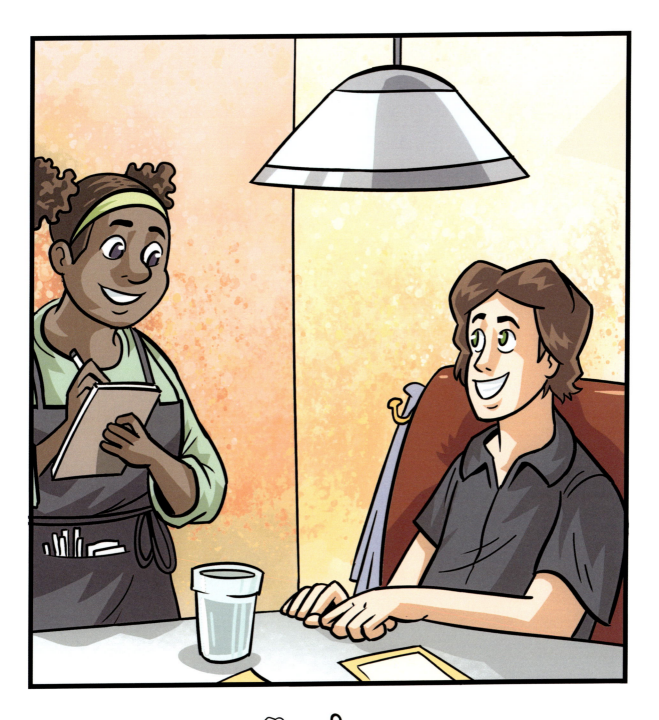

Would you like to order?

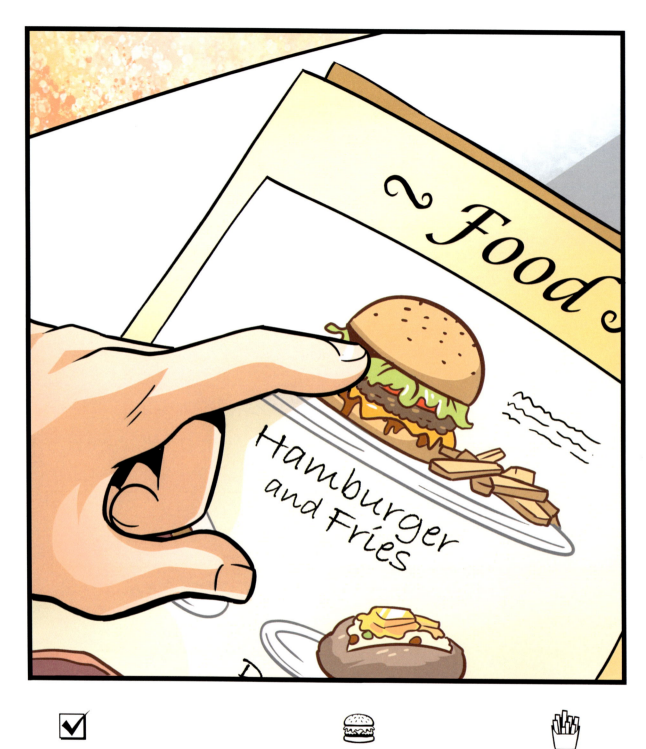

Yes, I'll have a hamburger and fries.

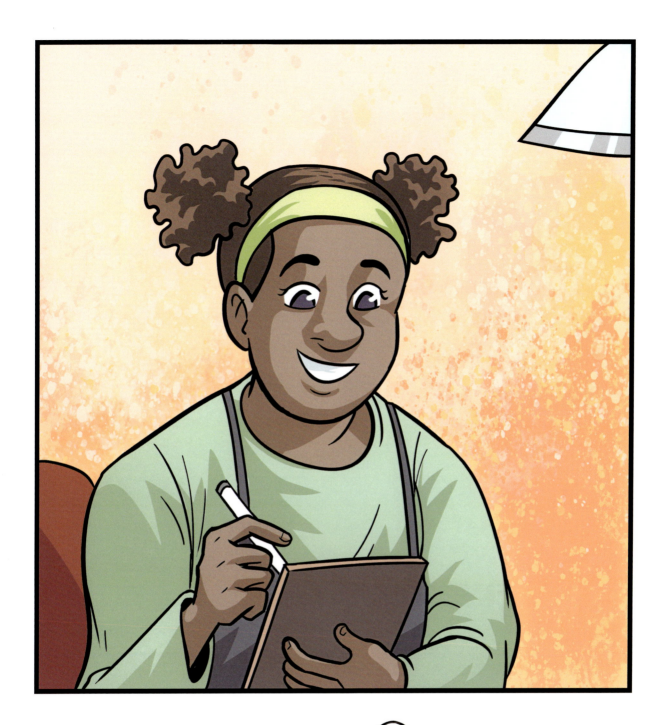

☺
Sounds good.

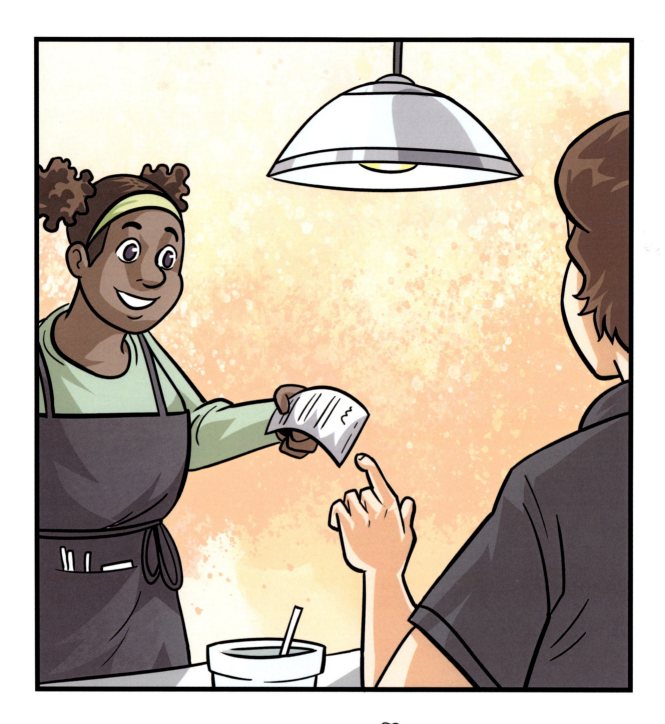

Thank you!

Customize and Practice Your Order

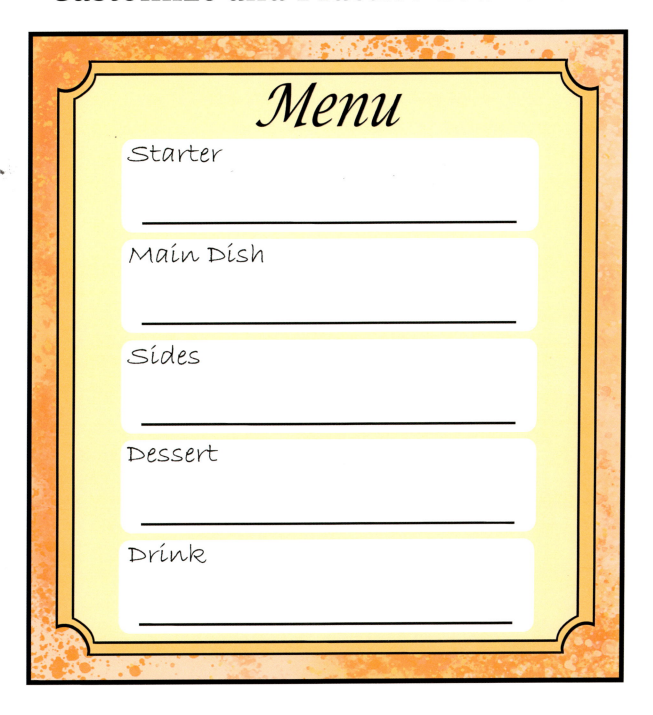

Notes

ACKNOWLEDGMENTS

Thank you to our family and friends, without which this dream would have never become a reality. We also thank our friends at the University of Michigan Aphasia Program at the University Center for Language and Literacy for their unyielding support of this passion project.

ABOUT THE AUTHOR

Anna Teal is a wife to her beloved husband, Ryan, and a passionate advocate for those fighting to overcome aphasia and apraxia. She owns her own copywriting business, Teal Marketing, LLC, and writes for various local magazines to share inspiring stories in her community. Anna's faith in God is a testament to her positive outlook and hope for a more meaningful life in light of tragic circumstances.